INTERMITTENT FASTING STUDIES

How Does Intermittent Fasting Work?

Copyright © 2019 Jill Sander

Table of Contents

INTRODUCTION

Intermittent fasting involves alternating festival times and hunger, during which you may eat whatever you want, but only drink water during the fast. The goal is to achieve the advantages of reducing calories and use it as a tool to lose weight for some.

Intermittent fasting may take place over several days, alternating 24 hours or daily periods. The first option requires that you abstain on one or more days of the week from particular or all meals. Regular fasting uses 24-hour lunch and fasting periods, starting at the same time every day, eating from Tuesday 6:00 to Wednesday 6:00from Monday 6:00, for example, to Tuesday 6:00, and repeating the process. There is a limited time to eat during intermittent fasting every day, usually four-six hours, in the 24-hour period during which you can consume as much as you want.

Some of the things that put people off are the fear that they will be starving and will not adhere to the plan or know-how. This is very easy if you plan that you eat your evening meal at about the same time each day, but at one hour on either side, depending on whether your meal is intermittent or food. Once, with a little preparation, you can also feed and socialize.

The main factor that prevents many people from trying is the fear of starvation. Although it takes a bit of willpower and a little discomfort to start with, it's quite simple!

CHAPTER ONE

Intermittent Fasting

Intermittent fasting (IF) leads to dietary eating patterns that do not consume or reduce calories excessively for some time. There are also many separate subgroups of intermittent fasting with specific duration variations, some for days, some for hours. This has become a popular subject in the scientific community because of all the potential fitness and health benefits discovered.

Fasting or periods of voluntary food withdrawal have been practiced worldwide for ages. Intermittent fasting to improve relatively new health. Intermittent fasting means restricting the intake of food for a certain period and does not affect the specific foods that you consume. Currently, the most common IF protocols are a 16 hour fast and a full day fasting, one or two days a week. Intermittent fasting could be regarded as a natural eating pattern in which humans were programmed to use and trace our Paleolithic ancestors. The current model of a proposed periodic fasting program, from body composition to longevity and aging, will help to improve many aspects of health. While IF goes against the norms of our community and traditional day-to-day routine, science may point to less frequency and faster time as the ideal solution for ordinary breakfast, lunch, and dinner template.

Here are two common myths about intermittent fasting.

Myth 1–You should eat three meals a day: this traditional "rule" in Western society was not developed based on health facts but was taken as the standard pattern for the colonists and gradually became the norm. In addition to the lack of scientific justification for the three meals a day method, recent studies may demonstrate that fewer foods and faster are best suited for human health. One study showed that the same amount of calories per day is better at one meal than three meals per day for weight loss and body composition. This finding is a fundamental concept that is extrapolated into intermittent rapidity, and if you decide to eat 1-2 meals a day, you may find it best.

Myth 2: You need breakfast; this is the biggest meal of the day: there are many false claims concerning the absolute necessity of daily breakfast. "Breakfast increases your metabolism" and "Food intake reduces later in the day" are the most common claims. These claims were denied and studied for 16 weeks with results that show no reduction in metabolism when skipping breakfast and no increase in food consumption at lunch and dinner. Intermittent fasting protocols can still be done while eating breakfast, but some people find it easier to eat or skip a late morning, and this common myth should not be inhibited.

FASTING TYPES:

Intermittent fasting takes different forms, and each can have a particular set of unique advantages. Each type of intermittent rapidity changes the speed-to-eat ratio. The benefits and effectiveness of these various protocols may differ on a case-by-case basis, and determine which one is best for you is essential. Factors that can influence which one you choose include health objectives, daily schedule, and current health status. Other days, time-constrained feeding, and modified fasting are the most common types of IF.

1. Alternate Day Fasting: This approach includes alternating days with no calories (food or beverages) and days of free food and food, whatever you want.

This plan has shown that it supports weight loss, improves blood cholesterol and fat levels, and improves blood inflammation markers.

The main downfall with this kind of intermittent fasting is because of reported hunger during fasting days that it is the hardest to keep up with.

2. Modified fasting is a protocol with scheduled fasting days, but fasting days permit a certain

amount of food. Generally, 20-25% of regular calories are allowed for fasting days; therefore, if you usually eat 2,000 calories on a regular day, you are allowed 400-500 calories on fasting days. The 5:2 part of this diet refers to the non-fasting to fasting days' ratio. You would generally eat in this diet for five consecutive days, then quickly or limit calories to 20-25 percent over two consecutive days.

This protocol is ideal for weight loss, body composition, and can also benefit blood sugar, lipids, and inflammation regulation. Research has demonstrated the effect of the 5:2 protocol to reduce weight loss, improve/lower blood inflammation markers (3), and show trending signs of improvements in insulin resistance. This modified 5:2 fasting diet led to decreased fat in animal studies, reduced hunger hormones (leptin), and increased protein levels that are responsible for fat burning and blood sugar regulation (adiponectin).

Modification of fasting 6:3 protocol is easy to follow and has a few adverse side effects, including hunger, low energy, and irritability. In contrast, studies have also seen improvements, such as reduced tension, reduced anger, lower fatigue, improved self-confidence, and a more positive mood.

3. Time-Restricted Eating: If you meet anyone who claims they are fasting intermittently; the chances

are that they are feeding time-restrictedly. This is a type of intermittent fasting which is used every day and involves only a small amount of calories and the rest of the day. Regular fasting periods in time-restricted feeding can range from 12-20 hours and 16/8 (fast for 16 hours, calorie intake for 8) is the most common method. The time of day is not essential for this protocol as long as you fast for a consecutive period and only eat within your permitted time frame. For instance, a person may eat his first meal at 7 pm in a 16/8 time-restricted feeding schedule and last meal at 3 pm (almost 3-7afternoon), while a person can eat his first meal at 1 pm and the last one at 10 pm (nearly 10-2 pm). This procedure is meant to be done every day and is very versatile, as long as you stay in a fasting/eating window.

Time-restricted feeding is one of the most straight-forward strategies to adopt. This can lead to optimal metabolic activity by using it with your daily work and sleep schedule. Time-restricted feeding is a great program for weight loss and improvements in body composition and some other health benefits. The few studies conducted in humans noted significant weight loss, decreases in fasting blood glucose and cholesterol improvements with no perceived changes in tension, depression, cold, fatigue, or confusion. Animal studies showed other preliminary results with time-constrained feeding to protect from obesity, high levels of insulin, fatty hepatic disease, and inflammation.

The easy application and promising results of time-restricted feeding can make it an excellent way to prevent/manage weight loss and chronic disease. It can be useful to start with lower fasting to eating ratio like 12/12 hours when implementing this protocol and finally to work up to 16/8 hours.

Beginners Intermittent Fasting

There are two rules to be followed by intermittent fasting:

(1) Fasting should be fun and NOT stressful.

(2) Fasting must be straightforward and NOT rigid.

From a more mature point of view, tips for intermittent fasting beginners. For those choosing to do intermittent fasting (IF), there are two main reasons: weight loss or wellbeing or both. It is, however, good to keep these two formulas: more rules= more complicated= less chance of succeeding In terms of health, a 24-hour off-dinner time is excellent, it significantly reduces your calorie intake without sacrificing what you want to eat in non-fast days, and perhaps even more importantly it stimulates your body to produce m Sure, that's the right growth hormone, the same one that you learn about famous people ' staying young.' The growth hormone has many anti-aging benefits, and the fat burning is among the most interesting!

How do I fast intermittently?

Ideally, 2 24-hour fasts in a week will be sufficiently good to offer significant health and weight loss benefits. Nonetheless, beginning with a 24-hour fast is not recommended for beginners except if you are entirely sure that you can do this.

There is no default IF law. Only try it and get it to work for you. Let your motto be simplicity and flexibility. Don't find yourself uncomfortable.

As a beginner, you "clear your minds from any other methods of weight loss and concentrate on IF." This is your first step to the success of IF. Just think about how often breakfast is an essential meal in a day, or you have to eat 6 to 10 small meals a day to lose weight. Stick with them if these laws work for you. But if you set your feet on an alternate speed route, it's better to put these concepts aside for at least the time you try IF.

Ready for your IF mindset? Then start with' skip meal' and see how your body reacts. This is the most straightforward and most natural way to begin your intermittent fasting journey.

Pick a day to try' skip breakfast.' Alternatively, they have milk, fresh juice, or coffee. Please do not have coffee. If that goes well, try' skip lunch' and move on. Anyone with a right fasting mentality can do a 24 hour fast. One good tip is not to think about food. Avoid social discussion in the pantry during lunchtime. Go on a walk or do a few simple exercises.

• Ignore the unplanted meal as far as it is normal and

does not interfere with your daily work;

• Early and late, i.e., ignore lunch;

• One meal a day, preferably for dinner only when you are comfortable and have time for enjoying a real meal.

An Understanding Into Intermittent Fasting and Its Benefits

Intermittent fasting is now quite a phenomenon. Recent studies have shown that people who tried to lose weight, health, and a long life expectancy have gone up. Serial rape is generally an eating pattern that alternates between periods of abstinence, which usually consume only food and not fasting. In other meanings, for the next 24 hours, a man or woman may eat anything he wants quickly. Science, religious, and cultural practices all over the world seem to support this method to weight control. Adherents of intermittent fasting claim that this is a way of becoming more careful about food.

There are many different fasts and hundreds of possible variations. Two types of intermittent fasts are the most essential and often used. First of all, there is the daily fast in which a person eats only every 20-28 hours in 4 hours. The second is to fast 1-3 times a week, also called alternate day fasting, during which a person will eat anything he wants one day and quickly all day long.

Intermittent fasting has many positive effects on animals, such as rodents and primates. One study shows that "the serum glucose and insulin levels have been reduced, and neurons have increased resistance to excitotoxic stress." In 2008, an intermittent fasting study showed that the lifespan in C rose by 40.4% and by 56.6%. Alternative day elegant (24 hours) and2-on-3 days (48 hours) of fasting in comparison with the ad libitum diets. And a 2009 study has shown that sporadic rat speeding improves long-term survival by pro-antigenic, anti-apoptotic, and anti-remodeling effects after chronic heart failure.

Scholars note that only a few studies of people practicing intermittent fasting have been performed. The influence on the body composition of exercise and meal frequency is an essential but mostly unexplored field of research. Nevertheless, some positive results have been obtained. Last month, a result was published in the Proceedings of the National Academy of sciences showing that calorie reduction 30 percent a day increases the older people's memory.

Intermittent Fasting Allows Your Body to Do the Work it Was Meant to Do

In so many weight loss and health journals, Fasting has made the headlines. As the diet aid, it is ubiquitous to help lose the fatter you always seem to pick up. The body also has tasks that it does without our assistance. One of these functions is burning fat.

However, intermittent fasting gives your body some push with the burning fat function. Eventually, the body knows how to consume a great deal of fat in a short time. Intermittent means fasting, no food, and only drinking water for a total of 24 hours. As crazy as it may seem, people, Intermittent Fasting has been very successful in reducing weight for many and feeling better in general. Intermittent rapidity helps our bodies quickly burn fat in several ways.

The role of hormones in the bodies is essential. Each hormone has its performance and function. It is our growth hormone that helps us burn fat. When we fast, our growth hormone starts working at a much faster rate to burn the fat over time. Fasting also brings our price of insulin down, so that we consume the fat in the body rather than store it.

For our hormones to burn fat, they must also use fat-burning enzymes. The two most critical fat-burning proteins are adipose tissue HSL and Muscle tissue LPL. HSL supports the body to release fat and transform it into energy and muscles, whereas LPL helps cells in our muscles to store fat to burn it as fuel. These enzymes help hormones burn fat twice as quickly when they work together. Through intermittent quacking, these hormones and enzymes can soon burn fat on a fast day.

Fasting is a great way to maintain a healthy and clean body and mind. Many people who regularly practice intermittent fasting claim that they have learned a lot about the way they eat. What is behind this is that they always think about food and what food they want on their fasting days. A stage of adrenaline produced by the body also increases during low-term Fasting, which makes your body fat and overdrive works twice as hard. Combine this with your increased metabolism and see how intermittent rapid weight loss is so common.

CHAPTER TWO

Intermittent Fasting System

A diet you adopt during intermittent fasting depends on the results you want and from which you also continue, so take a look and ask yourself: what do I want from it?

If you like to reduce your weight, but if you're going to lose some pounds to the beach, you have to take a closer look at your diet, then you may find that you can do that with a couple of weeks of intermittent fasting.

Even if you can do intermittent fasting in several different ways, we're just looking at a 24-hour fast, which can lose 27 pounds over two months. The primary approach is to spend 24 hours twice a week quickly, and it makes sense to do so a few days apart, and it is easier to spot one day when you are busy so that you are not distracted by hunger. At first, you may encounter desire, but these will occur, and you may find that hunger feelings no longer have a problem as you become more used to intermittent fasting. You can see that you are focused and concentrated when fasting, which is the opposite of what you expect, but many people experience it.

You can and should drink plenty of water during fasting to prevent dehydration; tea and coffee will be okay in as much you take only a blow of milk. If you're concerned that you don't get plenty of nutrients in your body, you might think of a celery, broccoli, ginger, and lime juice that tastes great and gets the rich nutrients into your body although it would be best to keep to milk, tea, and coffee if you could handle it.

Whether you're healthy or not, after three weeks of intermittent fasting, you should see a loss of weight and don't be discouraged when you don't realize much progress first; it's not a race and better to lose weight linearly over time instead of crashing down a few pounds. You're going to put this right back on. You may want to check your diet on non-fasting days and cut out high-sugar foods and any junk you usually eat after the first month. It has been found that sporadic fasting tends to make you want to eat healthier food freely.

If you are rapidly building a body, you might want to look at your macronutrients and learn how much protein and carbohydrates you have to eat, and that is much harder. You can find information on several websites that you have to spend time looking for the best results.

There are many advantages to intermittent fasting, some of which are more less wind, a general feeling of wellness, and a clearer mind. After a fasting period, it is crucial not to succumb to any temptation to binge eat, as this will reverse the benefit from intermittent fasting.

In the end, just by pursuing an intermittent fasting regimen for a couple of weeks two times a week, you can lose weight; you can lose more weight and if you stick to that program, but if you can change your diet in the days you don't eat, you can keep your weight off without resorting to failed diets or diets.

Intermittent Fasting Benefits

Everyone is always wondering what the next big secret of a diet is... In particular, people want to burn fat and build muscle while making the smallest possible effort. They want everything, and that's a little too much sometimes, lastly, with most programs.

But what if the whole industry were told that programs were ahead of it? Join Intermittent Fasting.

Let's kill a very perpetuated myth before we get to the benefits of intermittent Fasting.

Breakfast is the biggest meal of the day:

Those who participate regularly (often from sleep to lunch, which means skipping breakfast) report increasing focus, increased energy levels, and also a good mood as they are swift. Were you looking for your latest coffee? You have found one that gives you energy and burns fat.

Eating six foods a day accelerates metabolism:

When you consume the same number of calories and have the equal distribution of macronutrients (mainly of protectin), eating sure calories and nutrients are almost zero between 6 and 1 meals. Because if you cut calories at the end of the day, there will be the same caloric shortage, and if you add calories, there will be the same excess!

And if there was a difference, you tended to believe it was in favor of the method of Fasting.

Through increasing the resistance to insulin, intermittent Fasting will ensure that the calories are driven into your muscles when you eat! And if you're not fasting, the increased adrenaline will give you fat and strength!

In the purest sense, intermittent Fasting rotates between eating periods and eating periods. Here are the following benefits, but the general reason behind intermittent Fasting is that many people react very well to a reduction in calories, in particular during a diet.

It allows for appetite regulation, resistance to insulin (read: muscle building), and more time to burn fat (increased adrenaline).

Methods:

You can quickly go through your sleep and into the evening, and then have a food window lasting a few hours. You would also have the learning at this time.

Or it could mean you wake up and eat a big meal, then quickly late in the day until the last lunch.

Be intelligent and efficient; select a program that results in practical and researched methods. Whatever your responsibility, but to squeeze the most results from any way you choose, study, and listen to your body.

Improved insulin sensitivity/nutrient portioning is an excellent way of building muscle without becoming fat!

Adrenaline/noradrenaline increased, which means more time spent burning fat!

Reduced appetite and hunger, the possibility of feeling full by eating all calories in fewer meals. Example: Would you like to have 2900 calorie meals or 6300 calories meals if you are given 1,800 calories on your diet?

Energy and focus increased and so much more...

That's all you want in a diet. We want to take more advantage of the body of our dreams, and this is a perfect way! This is how you reach the fitness industry's number one target... Burning fat during muscle building!

The rest of the industry is far ahead of Intermittent Fasting. It contradicts many of the mainstream myths that you might believe are being perpetuated. We should then again, tell ourselves, again, do we want mainstream results? Or would we like to be more than average, unique, and top?

The Truth About Fasting

The advantages of fasting are great news lately. How successful is it, however? Some people are interested in it as a weight-loss tool, but it has many benefits over and above weight loss, and you can lose weight with it, some of which are very impressive. For some years, it has been known that it dramatically extends mice, and flies and worms even seem to prolong the lives of monkeys. Does it prolong human life? Many people are convinced, but the truth is we're still uncertain, also if it seems hopeful.

Nevertheless, it has medical benefits regarding cancer, cardiac disease, dementia, and even mood and well-being. It cannot be called a cure, but it lays the foundation for healing through the rest and recovery of vital parts of your body. There is no doubt that excess food places a burden on your body and sometimes requires rest. Besides, studies show that if it does not rest, much of the repair and regeneration necessary for optimal health is forgotten.

Glucose, Glycogen, and Fat

Your body needs the power to function correctly, and this energy is derived from the food you eat. Food is converted into a glucose form of sugar. Your cells (especially those in your brain) need a constant supply of glucose, and you start to feel weak and tired if it gets low.

After you eat, glucose circulates in your blood and is consumed quite quickly as you do your everyday tasks. If not refilled, it will potentially be drained in a few hours. This creates a problem: how do you keep your supply reasonable? Glucose alone cannot be stored but can be transformed into a form called glycogen, which can be saved in your muscles and liver. It can be drawn from here and used as needed. It's usually good for approximately 10 to 12 hours.

When it's depleted, what happens? Then the body turns to the fat cells stored all over your body. They can be broken down and transformed into ketones. This, of course, is what dietitians are seeking, namely the loss of fat cells. But you have to be careful if you stay too long in this point. The body soon begins to break down the protein; a rather complicated process can also convert it to glucose. And this causes muscle loss-something that you don't want. A fair amount of weight loss in most diets is caused by a loss of muscle along with water depletion (leaving you dehydrated). Don't be fooled. Don't be misled.

As noted earlier, you may lose weight by fasting, but most doctors and dieticians do not recommend long fasting periods as they can adversely impact your overall health. Weight loss by fasting.

However, it is hard for most people to quickly for long periods. A better alternative is what we call intermittent fasting when you usually rapidly eat on the other days of the week. One form of this is swiftness during the day. In that case, one day, you immediately (or limit your calories) and usually eat the next day. This works well for some people, but BBC's Dr. Michael Mosley proposed what he calls a 5-2 fasting diet. You limit your calories to only two days a week in this diet. These days, he suggests 600 calories for women and 700 for men. For most people, this is much easier, and it appears to produce the same results as wider fasts. Yet weight loss is not the most crucial advantage of such a diet, so look at the other benefits.

Health benefits of intermittent fasting It can be hard to believe, but intermittent fasting has tremendous benefits. The main thing it does is sit on many of the body's vital parts and organs to boost their function. Some of the following are:

- The digestive system rests. In effect, it benefits many other body parts.
- Reduces sugar in the blood. This reduces insulin production and makes it more reactive and active. Also, the pancreas rests.
- Regulated high blood pressure.
- Detoxification takes place. Fasting helps clear and detoxify your body. It is important to take enough water plenty of water for

this.
- This increases your strength and enhances your feeling.
- It helps protect you from heart and stroke disease.
- This helps reinvigorate the immune system and therefore battles chronic inflammation.
- Reduces oxidative stress in your cells caused by free radicals.

One of the hormones in the body is known as IGF-1 (insulin-like growth factor 1); it allows the cells to grow and is particularly important when it comes to raising children. Nevertheless, when you reach adulthood, it declines significantly. This is important because it appears to have adverse consequences as you get older: it accelerates aging and can even cause cancer. So when you're older, it's not something you want to be significant. Yet tests have shown that it reduces intermittent fasting.

A protein known as BDNF (brain-derived neurotrophic factor) is also found in your brain. This is significant because stem cells have been shown to turn into new neurons. The effects of BDNF arise in a brain section called the hippocampus, which is essential for memory and learning; it tends to protect against dementia and Alzheimer's disease and functions as an antidepressant, reducing anxiety.

Eventually, intermittent fasting leads to increased autophagy, a process in cells that destroys damaged molecules that may lead to severe neurological conditions.

Diabetes

Diabetes is diagnosed in two forms: diabetes I and diabetes II. Both cells use glucose as energy, as we saw earlier. But without glucose, it can't get into the cells. Insulin is formed employing the blood glucose quantity in the pancreas; the function is to permit glucose to reach the cavity. A lot of cells in the body have insulin receptors, which bind to insulin, which circulates in your blood. If insulin is attached to the surface of a cell, it allows glucose in, so it plays an integral part in your body. However, too much can be harmful. Insulin increases your starvation, helps fat cell storage, and is associated with diabetes and heart problems.

One of the significant insulin problems is what is known as insulin resistance. In this situation, insulin is produced by the pancreas, but insulin receptors no longer work properly on the cells and do not allow glucose to enter as it should be. Glucose begins to accumulate in the blood without a place to go, and the cells start to die early. In an attempt to get sucrose into the cells, the body knows that something is wrong, and the pancreas releases more insulin, but it does cause the pancreas overwork and eventually starts wearing out. Diabetes II is the result.

Studies have shown that intermittent quickness improves your sensitivity to insulin. This, in turn, allows your body to control blood glucose levels better after meals and thus helps restore your pancreas. Both are important in terms of diabetes II prevention.

The fasting rules

- A 5-2 method is recommended, with regular meals five days a week and with limited food for two days (500 calories for females, 600 calories for males).
- Stay hydrated. Stay hydrated. Drink abundant water; it helps to flush out toxins.
- If you do not fast (and even fast), keep your nutrition maximized.
- Especially eat enough vegetables, fruits, and whole grains.
- Note that the impact requires 12 hours of fasting. It's best for 12 to 18 hours. It is above 18. It is beyond 18.
- You can exercise, but don't overdo it during fasting periods.
- Be careful when you're diabetic to fast.

3 Tips to Make Intermittent Fasting Easier

The Carb Contact One of the most significant factors to determine the ease of your speed is your fast food's carbohydrates content. The high consumption of carbon the day before a quick day will dramatically increase my hunger and hunger during a fast period. The faster my carb consumption goes, the easier, the faster it looks.

Enhancement as compared to the real or physiological needs for nutrients and heat. Fasting is one of the best ways to learn the difference between the two since the qualities of hunger are known. Hormonal desire is, however, the result of the interplay of different hormones in your body, regardless of physiological needs.

hormonal starvation: "Hormonal hunger emerges from significant fluctuation in insulin rate and is responsible for extreme hunger pangs and wild, unreasonable cravings that can even overwhelm the most determined dietary material. Insulin naturally ebbs and flows under dynamic pressure with glucagon. But the important message here is that hormones are all played and triggered by catalysts, like the foods you are eating. If you give one of your hormones a massive stimulus–like throwing sugar into insulin–you can imagine you can start a flow of hormonal imbalance, which can last for many hours (if not days).

You can think of it like putting a ruthless child with a bunch of quiet children in a room. The loud one riles up the others and sets off the entire room. And even when the original wild child begins to get tired or windy, the others are going to reverse him or her.

Once you get your hormones revived and bounce off like this, it takes a while to get them cooked down to the point where hormonal starvation is normalized, and real hunger is felt.

3 Tips to make quicker:

1. Do not eat much before your fast begins.

Especially when you begin using Intermittent Fasting, it can be very tenting to pick up quickly. This is part of the psychological fear of "starving," which the food industry has strengthened. But a big meal before beginning your fast, regardless of the macronutrient composition, will set off that hormonal imbalance that we try to prevent.

2. Always avoid processed white sugar before you quickly.

But you might also like to consider reducing other

sources of simple sugars, like dried fruit, high GI fruits, like bananas and milk, before your fast. All of these tend to rub your hormones.

3. Try to prevent starchy carbs like hot sweet potato, some succulent butterfly squash.

Still, before you get quick, or gentle steel-cut oatmeal has nothing right, it can be a stimulant enough to release insulin that can make your fasting Hormonal Hunger more prominent. Try to avoid grains and potatoes most of the time, but don't touch them with a ten-foot pole beforehand. And, of course, all processed foodstuffs made from a white meal should at any time be minimized.

So what can you eat in front of your fast? The staples should be protein, good fats, and veggies. The menu might include beef, pork, bison, shrimp, turkey, lamb, broccoli, chocolate, salad, spinach, tomato, pepper, green olive oil, coconut oil, etc. This list is, of course, very incomplete, but it gives you the idea. You can pay it off as long as it's on similar lines as you like.

CONCLUSION

Intermittent fasting is an alternating controlled fasting pattern. Fasting? Does "not eat" mean? Yes, mean not to eat. Some of us chow down on food we can take when we are hungry. It includes junk foods, processed foods, and fast foods most of the time. We see fast food everywhere we go. We see street food everywhere we go, and so on. We eat three food a day, as well as three meals, which are not enough for some of us yet. Each time we feel hungry, or every time we feel the need for the food, we tend to feed ourselves more. We know very well that this is right, but we don't think of it, and we try to give in.

Only breakfast, lunch, and dinner are daily meals. These are the only foods that matter to us. All other meals are extra and usually not necessary, which leads us to add our weight and produce fat. If we don't work too much and physical activity takes place most of the time, we could also feed on hunger. Because if we don't do much physical activity, we should not give in to this tempting desire.

So what are we doing?

That's when we eat our daily meals in one day and run for the next 24 hours. We don't necessarily mean you can't take anything into your belly. We want to have your drink in water or any healthy fruit juice. However, we recommend water is better.

Water in our body does a lot of good things. It purifies our body and helps to remove unhealthy food. Many scientific studies and research show that intermittent fasting is very beneficial to our health. Remember before that when our ancestors were hungry, they had no fast food, junk food, or street food. What do they do? What do they do? They drink water to lose their hunger. Most of the time, we feel a desire not because we are starving, but because our mind and body are reasonable to feed. This is what we call mental hunger. Sometimes we cheat our minds.

That's the tip for intermittent fasting. For instance, you can eat as much food today as you want. But be prepared to let you drink water for twenty-four hours after dinner tonight. Drink water as much as your hunger needs to feed. This process trains your mind and body not to allow you to eat when you don't have to eat. This fast leads your body to use the stored fat and energy that is not used for a long time. So you lose weight and stay healthier.

Intermittent fasting is not recommended for everyone. This is ideal only for those without health problems. Whenever you want to try intermittent fasting, you should consult your doctor in advance.

Thanks for reading.

www.ingramcontent.com/pod-product-compliance
Lightning Source LLC
Chambersburg PA
CBHW051426250726

48655CB00003B/1255